INTRODUCTION TO FASTING

Nicolas Joseph

Copyright © 2024 [Nicolas Joseph]

Disclaimer

First Edition: [August, 2024]

Printed in [USA]

____

Cover Design by [Nicolas Joseph]

Editing by [Nicolas Joseph]

Published by [Amazon]

https://kdp.amazon.com

Thank you for purchasing and reading this book. Your support allows us to continue to provide high-quality content. If you enjoyed this book, please consider leaving a review on Amazon.com. Your feedback is greatly appreciated.

____

INTRODUCTION

In a world where food is abundant and readily available, the practice of fasting might seem counterintuitive, even daunting. However, the concept of fasting from eating is as old as humanity itself, deeply rooted in various cultural, religious, and health traditions. This book explores the multifaceted world of fasting, delving into its significance, spiritual foundations, and contemporary applications.

Fasting is not merely an act of abstaining from food; it is a journey of self-discovery, discipline, and healing. Throughout history, people have embraced fasting for its physical benefits, such as detoxification and weight management, as well as for its mental and spiritual rewards, including clarity of thought, emotional resilience, and a heightened sense of purpose.

In recent years, scientific research has begun to catch up with what many ancient traditions have long understood: fasting can profoundly impact our health and well-being. From intermittent fasting to extended fasts, the evidence points to numerous benefits, including improved metabolic health, reduced inflammation, and enhanced longevity.

As you turn the pages, you will discover that fasting is not about deprivation but about renewal. It is an opportunity to reset your body, mind, and spirit, to break free from unhealthy habits, and to embrace a more mindful and intentional way of living. Welcome to the transformative world of fasting—a practice that has the power to change your life in profound and unexpected ways.

PART I: BENEFITS

Weight Loss

Fasting naturally leads to a reduction in calorie intake, as it involves skipping meals or eating within a restricted time window. By consuming fewer calories than the body requires to maintain its current weight, an energy deficit is created. This deficit forces the body to tap into stored fat reserves to meet its energy needs, leading to fat loss over time. For instance, intermittent fasting, where individuals might eat all their daily calories within a 6 to 8 hour window, often results in consuming fewer calories overall, even without intentional restriction.

When fasting, the body's insulin levels drop. Insulin is a hormone that regulates blood sugar levels and facilitates the storage of fat. Lower insulin levels encourage the body to burn fat for energy rather than relying on glucose from recent meals. During fasting periods, glycogen stores (the stored form of glucose) in the liver are depleted. Once these stores are low, the body begins to break down fat into fatty acids and ketones, which are then used as alternative energy sources. This state, known as ketosis, is particularly effective for fat burning and is a key reason why fasting can lead to weight loss.

Improved Insulin Sensitivity

Fasting has been shown to improve insulin sensitivity, which is the body's ability to effectively use insulin to regulate blood sugar levels. During fasting, insulin levels drop, allowing the body to rely on stored fat for energy instead of glucose. This shift reduces the demand for insulin, giving insulin receptors in the cells time to rest and reset.

Over time, this can lead to increased efficiency in how these receptors respond to insulin, thereby improving insulin sensitivity. Enhanced insulin sensitivity helps the body maintain more stable blood sugar levels, reducing the risk of insulin resistance and associated conditions like type 2 diabetes. Additionally, fasting reduces inflammation and oxidative stress, which are both factors that can impair insulin function.

Autophagy

Fasting stimulates autophagy, a cellular process where the body cleans out damaged cells and regenerates new, healthy ones. This process is vital for maintaining cellular health and function. By promoting the removal of dysfunctional cells and proteins, autophagy helps prevent diseases, including cancer and neurodegenerative disorders.

It also supports overall longevity and health by ensuring that cells function optimally. Beyond cellular cleanup, autophagy initiated by fasting has been linked to a lower risk of diseases such as Alzheimer's, Parkinson's, and Huntington's. This process helps clear out misfolded proteins and damaged organelles, which are associated with neurodegenerative diseases. Autophagy also supports the immune system by removing intracellular pathogens and promoting the recycling of cellular components.

Reduced Inflammation

Fasting can significantly reduce inflammation, which is linked to numerous chronic diseases such as heart disease, cancer, and arthritis. By lowering levels of inflammatory markers like C-reactive protein (CRP), fasting helps mitigate the risk of these conditions. Reduced inflammation also aids in the healing of existing injuries and the prevention of new inflammatory issues, contributing to overall health and wellness.

Chronic inflammation is a root cause of many diseases, and fasting can help by reducing the production of pro-inflammatory cytokines. Fasting induces a reduction in oxidative stress, which further decreases inflammation. This anti-inflammatory effect can improve symptoms of conditions such as rheumatoid arthritis, inflammatory bowel disease, and asthma, enhancing overall quality of life.

Heart Health

Fasting benefits heart health by improving several cardiovascular risk factors, including cholesterol levels, blood pressure, and triglycerides. By reducing LDL cholesterol (bad cholesterol) and increasing HDL cholesterol (good cholesterol), fasting helps prevent the buildup of plaque in arteries. Lower blood pressure and triglyceride levels further reduce the risk of heart disease and stroke, promoting a healthier cardiovascular system.

Fasting can lead to improved heart health by not only lowering cholesterol and triglyceride levels but also by reducing markers of inflammation such as interleukin-6 and C-reactive protein. This reduction in inflammation helps prevent the development of atherosclerosis, the buildup of fatty deposits in arteries, thereby reducing the risk of heart attacks and strokes.

Enhanced Brain Function

Fasting has been shown to improve brain function by increasing the production of brain-derived neurotrophic factor (BDNF), a protein that supports the growth and survival of neurons. It also stimulates the growth of new brain cells and enhances cognitive function, memory, and learning. Fasting may also protect against neurodegenerative diseases like Alzheimer's and Parkinson's by reducing inflammation and oxidative stress in the brain.

Fasting supports brain health by promoting the production of ketones, an efficient fuel for the brain. Ketones provide more energy per unit of oxygen compared to glucose, enhancing brain energy metabolism. Fasting also increases mitochondrial biogenesis in the brain, which boosts cognitive function and resilience against stress.

Improved Metabolic Health

Fasting can boost metabolic health by increasing levels of norepinephrine, a hormone that enhances metabolism and promotes fat burning. This increase in metabolic rate can help the body burn more calories even at rest, contributing to weight loss and improved energy balance. Fasting also helps regulate hormones involved in metabolism, such as leptin and ghrelin, which control hunger and satiety.

Fasting helps improve metabolic health by stabilizing blood sugar levels and reducing insulin resistance. This stabilization prevents the spikes and crashes associated with regular eating patterns, leading to more consistent energy levels.

Longevity

Research suggests that fasting can extend lifespan by promoting cellular repair, reducing inflammation, and enhancing metabolic health. By improving overall health and reducing the risk of age-related diseases, fasting can contribute to a longer and healthier life. The activation of autophagy and other cellular processes during fasting plays a crucial role in maintaining the body's function and vitality over time.

The potential longevity benefits of fasting are attributed to its ability to mimic calorie restriction, which has been shown to extend lifespan in various species. Fasting promotes stress resistance and reduces the incidence of age-related diseases by enhancing DNA repair mechanisms and reducing the accumulation of cellular damage, thereby promoting healthier aging.

Cancer Prevention

Fasting has been studied for its potential role in cancer prevention, with research suggesting that it can contribute to reducing the risk of cancer by promoting cellular repair and enhancing the body's natural defense mechanisms. During fasting, the body enters a state of autophagy, a process where damaged or dysfunctional cells are broken down and recycled. This not only helps in maintaining healthy cells but also reduces the likelihood of cellular mutations that could lead to cancer.

Additionally, fasting can lower insulin levels and reduce inflammation, both of which are associated with a decreased risk of cancer development. While fasting shows promise, it should be approached with caution and under medical guidance, particularly for individuals with existing health conditions.

Gut Health

Fasting can improve gut health by giving the digestive system a break, allowing it to reset and function more efficiently. This rest period helps promote a healthier balance of gut bacteria, which is essential for digestion, immunity, and overall health. Fasting may also reduce symptoms of digestive disorders like irritable bowel syndrome (IBS) and promote the healing of the gut lining.

Fasting promotes gut health by encouraging the growth of beneficial gut bacteria, which play a crucial role in digestion, immunity, and overall health. A healthier gut microbiome can improve nutrient absorption, reduce symptoms of gastrointestinal disorders, and enhance the gut-brain axis, which influences mood and cognitive function.

PART II: MORE?

Improved Immune System

Fasting strengthens the immune system by reducing inflammation and promoting the regeneration of immune cells. During fasting, the body shifts its focus to maintaining vital functions, which includes enhancing immune response. This can help protect against infections, reduce the severity of autoimmune conditions, and improve the body's ability to fight diseases.

Fasting enhances the immune system by stimulating the production of new white blood cells and reducing inflammation. This regeneration of immune cells improves the body's ability to fight infections and diseases. Fasting also helps clear out damaged and dysfunctional cells, reducing the risk of autoimmune diseases and chronic inflammation.

Better Skin Health:

Fasting can lead to clearer, healthier skin by reducing inflammation and promoting detoxification. Fasting helps the body eliminate toxins more efficiently, which can reduce skin issues like acne and eczema. Additionally, fasting-induced autophagy supports skin cell regeneration, leading to a more youthful appearance.

Fasting can improve skin health by reducing the occurrence of acne and other skin conditions linked to high insulin levels and inflammation. By stabilizing blood sugar and reducing inflammation, fasting helps maintain clearer, healthier skin. The detoxification process during fasting also promotes a more radiant complexion.

Improved Mental Clarity and Focus

Fasting can enhance cognitive function, mental clarity, and focus by optimizing brain function. The increase in BDNF and other neuroprotective factors during fasting supports brain health and cognitive performance. Many people report feeling more alert and focused during fasting periods, likely due to stabilized blood sugar levels and the brain's efficient use of ketones for energy.

The mental clarity and focus experienced during fasting are partly due to increased production of neurotrophic factors and improved synaptic plasticity. These changes enhance learning and memory processes. Additionally, fasting reduces brain fog often associated with high blood sugar levels, leading to sharper cognitive function and better decision-making.

Enhanced Detoxification

Fasting aids in detoxification by giving the liver and other detox organs a break, allowing them to function more efficiently. The reduction in food intake during fasting periods helps the body focus on eliminating accumulated toxins, which can improve overall health and reduce the risk of toxin-related diseases.

The detoxification benefits of fasting include the enhancement of the liver's ability to metabolize and eliminate toxins. Fasting increases the production of enzymes involved in detoxification processes, leading to more efficient toxin removal. This detoxification supports overall health by reducing the burden of harmful substances in the body.

Improved Digestive Efficiency

Fasting enhances the efficiency of the digestive system by giving it a rest from constant food processing. This break allows the digestive organs to repair and regenerate, leading to better nutrient absorption and overall digestive health.

It can also alleviate symptoms of digestive disorders and improve bowel regularity. This rest period helps reset the gut microbiota, promoting a healthy balance of beneficial bacteria. Improved digestive efficiency can alleviate symptoms of bloating, gas, and indigestion, leading to better overall digestive health.

Balanced Cholesterol Levels

During fasting, the body shifts its energy source from glucose to stored fats, which leads to a reduction in triglycerides, a type of fat linked to heart disease. This process also helps lower low-density lipoprotein (LDL), commonly known as "bad" cholesterol, which can accumulate in the arteries and increase the risk of cardiovascular issues.

At the same time, fasting can raise high-density lipoprotein (HDL), the "good" cholesterol, which helps remove excess cholesterol from the bloodstream. These changes collectively contribute to better overall cholesterol profiles, reducing the risk of heart disease and promoting cardiovascular health.

Boosted Energy Levels

Some people experience increased energy levels and reduced fatigue after fasting. This boost in energy is likely due to the body's improved efficiency in using energy stores and the stabilization of blood sugar levels. Enhanced metabolic function during fasting also contributes to sustained energy throughout the day.

The boost in energy levels during fasting is also due to improved mitochondrial function. Fasting enhances mitochondrial efficiency and biogenesis, leading to better energy production at the cellular level. This increase in cellular energy translates to higher physical and mental energy, reducing feelings of fatigue and sluggishness.

Lower Blood Pressure

Fasting can lead to a reduction in blood pressure, which lowers the risk of heart disease and stroke. By improving insulin sensitivity and reducing inflammation, fasting helps maintain healthy blood pressure levels, contributing to overall cardiovascular health.

Fasting helps lower blood pressure by reducing insulin resistance and improving arterial function. The reduction in insulin levels during fasting leads to decreased sodium retention, which lowers blood pressure. Improved endothelial function and reduced arterial stiffness further contribute to maintaining healthy blood pressure levels.

PART III: EVEN MORE

Improved Sleep

Fasting can help regulate sleep patterns and improve the quality of sleep, by reducing late-night eating and stabilizing blood sugar levels. Fasting supports the body's natural sleep-wake cycle, leading to more restful and restorative sleep.

The regulation of sleep patterns through fasting is supported by its impact on circadian rhythms. Fasting helps synchronize the body's internal clock, leading to more consistent sleep-wake cycles. Improved sleep quality enhances overall health, cognitive function, and mood, making fasting a beneficial practice for better sleep hygiene.

Enhanced Muscle Growth

Fasting can stimulate the production of growth hormone, which supports muscle growth and fat loss. This hormone is crucial for maintaining muscle mass, especially during weight loss, and for promoting overall physical fitness and strength.

The increase in growth hormone levels during fasting supports muscle growth by promoting protein synthesis and reducing muscle breakdown. This effect is particularly beneficial for athletes and individuals engaged in strength training. Fasting also enhances the body's ability to utilize fat for energy, preserving muscle mass during periods of caloric deficit.

Reduced Oxidative Stress

Fasting reduces oxidative stress by lowering the production of free radicals and enhancing the body's antioxidant defenses. This reduction in oxidative stress is vital for preventing cellular damage, aging, and the development of chronic diseases.

Fasting reduces oxidative stress by enhancing the production of antioxidant enzymes and reducing the generation of reactive oxygen species. This reduction in oxidative stress protects cells from damage, slows the aging process, and reduces the risk of chronic diseases associated with oxidative damage, such as cardiovascular disease and cancer.

Hormonal Balance

Fasting helps balance hormones like leptin and ghrelin, which regulate hunger and satiety. By stabilizing these hormones, fasting can reduce overeating, improve appetite control, and support healthy weight management. Fasting's impact on hormonal balance includes the regulation of thyroid hormones, which play a key role in metabolism and energy levels.

By stabilizing thyroid hormone levels, fasting supports better metabolic function and energy balance. Additionally, fasting helps balance sex hormones, which can improve reproductive health and reduce symptoms of hormonal imbalances.

Enhanced Fat Burning

Fasting shifts the body into a fat-burning mode by depleting glycogen stores and increasing lipolysis, the breakdown of fats for energy. This process promotes the efficient use of fat stores, leading to weight loss and improved body composition.

The shift to fat burning during fasting is supported by increased levels of adiponectin, a hormone that enhances fat metabolism. This shift not only promotes weight loss but also improves insulin sensitivity and reduces the risk of metabolic disorders. Enhanced fat burning also supports sustained energy levels and improved athletic performance.

Reduced Appetite

Fasting can help reduce appetite and cravings by stabilizing blood sugar levels and balancing hunger hormones. This effect makes it easier to adhere to a healthy diet and avoid overeating, supporting long-term weight management and health. The improved regulation of hunger hormones supports long-term dietary adherence and weight management.

Also fasting allows your body to get used to being without for a period without it being an issue, which is a good way to create a healthy food eating habit and not be reliant on food too much. There may come situations where food may not be available and it's good to know that not having food will not bring your daily life to a complete halt, at least for a good while.

Improved Mood

Some people experience improved mood and a

sense of well-being during and after fasting periods. The stabilization of blood sugar levels and the release of endorphins during fasting contribute to these positive mood changes, enhancing overall mental health.

The mood-enhancing effects of fasting are also linked to the stabilization of neurotransmitters such as serotonin and dopamine. By promoting a healthy balance of these neurotransmitters, fasting helps reduce symptoms of depression and anxiety. The reduction in inflammation and oxidative stress during fasting further supports improved mental health and emotional well-being.

Better Hydration

Better hydration through fasting may seem counterintuitive, but it can enhance the body's ability to regulate fluid balance. When fasting, the body shifts its focus from digesting food to more essential functions, including efficient water utilization and retention. Without the intake of food, which often contains dehydrating elements like salt and sugar, the kidneys can work more effectively to maintain optimal hydration levels.

Additionally, fasting periods often lead to increased water consumption as individuals replace food intake with fluids. This heightened awareness and consumption of water can improve overall hydration, support cellular functions, and promote better skin health, digestion, and energy levels. Therefore, incorporating mindful fasting practices, along with adequate water intake, can be a beneficial strategy for improving hydration and overall well-being.

Enhanced Physical Endurance

Fasting can improve endurance and performance in physical activities by optimizing energy utilization. The increased production of growth hormone and the shift to fat as a primary energy source during fasting enhance physical stamina and strength.

Fasting enhances physical endurance by improving the body's ability to utilize stored fat for energy, which provides a more sustainable energy source during prolonged physical activity. This increased reliance on fat stores reduces the depletion of glycogen, allowing for improved stamina and endurance during exercise and other physical activities.

Greater Appreciation for Food

Fasting creates a deeper appreciation for food by stripping away the constant availability that often leads to its underappreciation. When we fast, we temporarily remove food from our daily routine, making its absence felt more keenly.

This absence heightens our awareness of hunger and the satisfaction that comes with nourishing our bodies. As a result, when we finally break the fast, even simple meals taste richer, and we become more mindful of the flavors, textures, and the effort involved in preparing food. This renewed gratitude for food fosters a healthier relationship with eating, where food is not just a routine necessity but a valued experience.

Conclusion: Introduction to Fasting

As we reach the end of this journey into the world of fasting, it's clear that this ancient practice offers a wealth of benefits that extend far beyond mere weight loss. Fasting is a powerful tool that can help reset our bodies, enhance mental clarity, and promote longevity. By allowing our systems to take a break from constant digestion and refueling, we tap into a natural process that supports cellular repair, reduces inflammation, and balances hormones.

But fasting is not just about physical health. The mental and spiritual aspects of fasting—whether through improved focus, a deeper sense of mindfulness, or a renewed connection to our body's signals—play an equally important role. By learning to listen to our bodies and embracing periods of rest, we cultivate a greater sense of self-awareness and resilience.

It's important to remember that fasting is a personal journey. What works for one person may not work for another, and it's essential to approach fasting with flexibility, understanding, and respect for our own unique needs. Consulting with healthcare professionals, experimenting with different fasting methods, and paying attention to our body's responses are crucial steps to ensure that fasting enhances, rather than detracts from, our overall well-being.

In a world where we're constantly bombarded with food and often disconnected from our body's natural rhythms, fasting offers a return to simplicity—a way to realign with our innate health and vitality. Whether you're seeking to improve your health, sharpen your mind, or simply reconnect with your body, fasting can be a powerful ally on your journey to a more balanced and vibrant life.

As you move forward, may you find the fasting approach that suits you best, and may it bring you the health, clarity, and inner peace you seek. Remember, the journey of fasting is not just about abstaining from food; it's about nourishing your body, mind, and spirit in new and profound ways.

Thank you.

A b o u t   t h e   A u t h o r

I am a happily married husband and father, who also has a deep love for health and fitness. Born in Haiti and raised there until the age of 13, I always understood the importance of taking care of your body being that you only get one. It wasn't until I came to the USA that I started to understand just how good and valuable eating food that has nutritional value is since back home I had it all natural and organic. As I began to learn more about the effects of nutrition depleted foods and their negative effects on the body, I started to investigate how I can help my body to repair itself from the unknowing damages that I have done to it. Wonderfully enough I stumbled unto fasting and the different types, and after learning more about the topic I realized how amazing the benefits were.

It is that love and appreciation that has motivated me to write this book, and this is of course but an introduction to the world of fasting. In the following series I will go over the types of fasting and help you to determine which one is best for you if you decide to give it a try. See you in the next chapter.

REFERENCES

Healthline. (n.d.). *8 health benefits of fasting,*

backed by science. Healthline. Retrieved August 28, 2024, from https://www.healthline.com/nutrition/fasting-benefits

Global Healing. (2023, March 16). *The health benefits of fasting*. Global Healing. Retrieved August 28, 2024, from https://explore.globalhealing.com/health-benefits-of-fasting

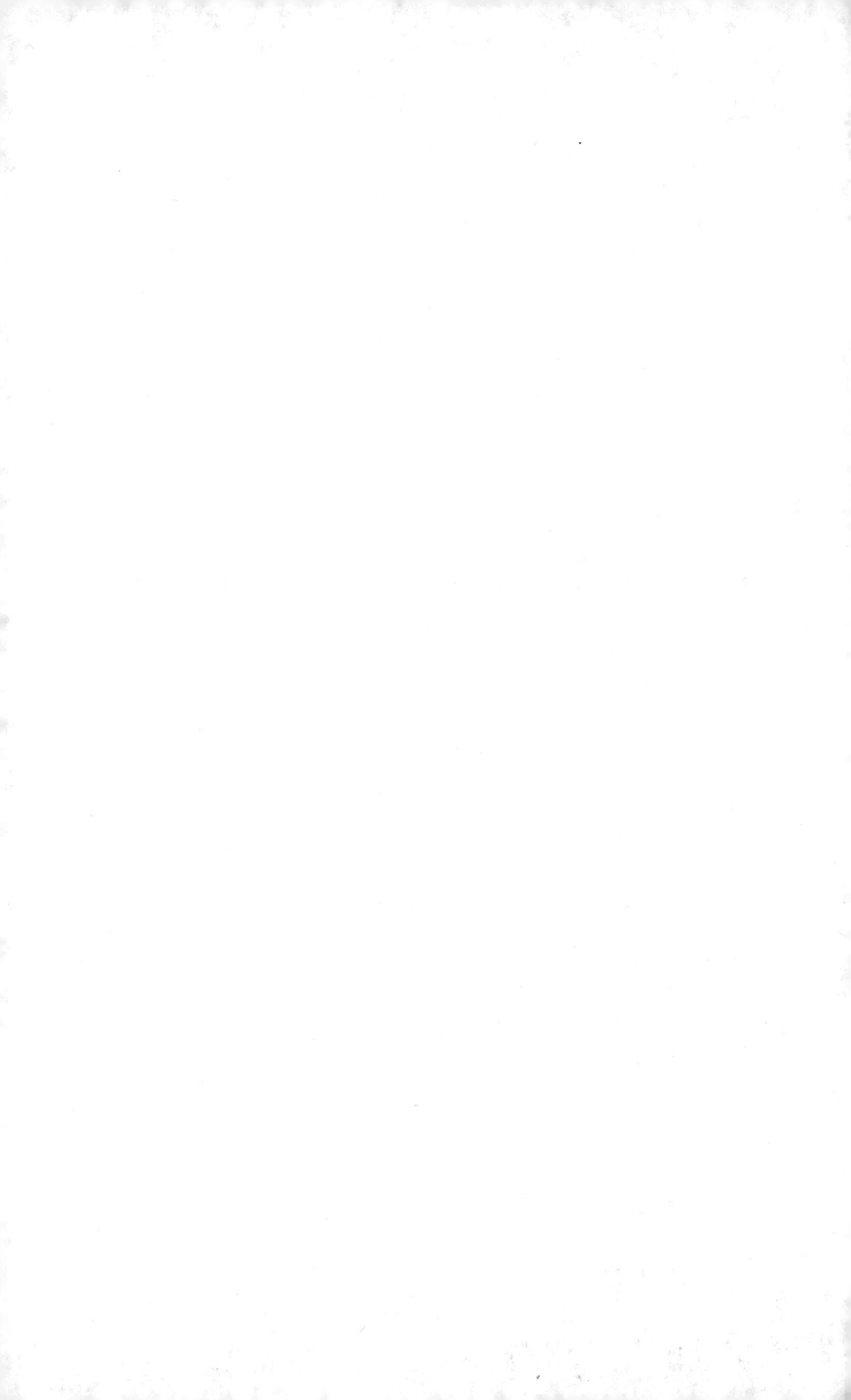